HERBAL REMEDIES FOR PAIN RELIEF AND SLEEP AID

Discover Natural Healing On Targeted Restful Sleep For Holistic Wellness, Vibrant Health And Happier Life

DR. CARDEN KYRIE

DISCLAIMER

The only goal of this book is informational. Every effort has been taken by the author and publisher to ensure that the information provided is accurate. But the material in this book is given "as is," without any express or implied representation, warranty, or condition as to its accuracy, completeness, or suitability for any particular purpose.

Any loss, damage, or injury resulting from using the information in this book, or from any action or decision made as a result of such use, will not be covered by the author's or publisher's liability. It is recommended that readers seek the assistance of a certified specialist for guidance specific to their situation.

The opinions and viewpoints conveyed in this book belong to the author and may not necessarily represent the official stance or policies of any specified organizations or people. Any likeness to real-life occurrences, places, or people—living or deceased—is wholly coincidental.

No specific product, service, or therapy discussed in this book is endorsed by the author or publisher. Any reference to goods or services is made only for informative reasons and is not intended as a recommendation or endorsement.

Before making any judgments or acting on any information, readers are urged to independently confirm it all. Any unfavorable effects or repercussions arising from the usage of the material included in this book are disclaimed by the author and publisher.

By using this book, you consent to absolving the publisher and author of any and all claims, obligations, or losses resulting from your use of the material in it.

I appreciate your cooperation and understanding.

TABLE OF CONTENTS

CHAPTER ONE

INTRODUCTION TO PAIN RELIEF AND SLEEP AID

Herbal treatments for a range of health issues have seen a noticeable upsurge in popularity in recent years, especially when it comes to pain management and sleep help. The attraction of herbal substitutes is their ability to provide medicinal advantages with fewer adverse effects in comparison to traditional medications. This move toward the use of herbal remedies is indicative of a heightened understanding of the holistic approach to health and the complex relationship that exists between the body and the environment. In this overview, we explore the many advantages of using herbal remedies for pain and sleeplessness and look at the special qualities they offer. A quick rundown of herbal treatments also gives a context-rich understanding of the cultural and historical foundations of the usage of plants for therapeutic purposes.

HERBAL PAIN RELIEF AND SLEEP AID BENEFITS

The emphasis on natural substances produced from plants is one of the main draws of herbal pain relief and sleep aids. These substances frequently cooperate to provide the body with a comprehensive and well-rounded effect. Herbal medicines are typically seen to be gentler and less likely to cause unpleasant responses than some synthetic medications. Herbs having anti-inflammatory qualities, such as turmeric, ginger, and boswellia, may help relieve pain without posing the same risks to the heart and digestive systems as prolonged use of some medications.

Herbs with relaxing and sedative properties, like passionflower, chamomile, and valerian root, have become increasingly popular as sleep aids. These plants have the potential to help control sleep cycles without having the side effects or grogginess that come with some prescription sleep aids. Some herbs, including ashwagandha, have adaptogenic properties that can lower stress levels generally and encourage a calm, sleep-inducing state.

Herbal therapies for pain reduction and sleep aid frequently address the underlying causes of suffering in addition to their physiological benefits. Herbs may address the underlying cause of a problem, as opposed to pharmaceuticals that only cover up symptoms, to support long-term health. This all-encompassing strategy is in line with the increasing societal movement towards self-care and preventative healthcare, which emphasizes general health rather than just treating specific symptoms.

A SYNOPSIS OF HERBAL TREATMENTS

Herbal medicines have their roots in ancient cultures when people learned via trial and error about the medicinal qualities of plants. Herbal medicine has a long history of use in many different cultures, including Traditional Chinese Medicine and Ayurveda in India. Herbal medicine's knowledge and insight have been handed down through the ages, creating a wealth of botanical understanding.

A vast variety of plants, each with a distinct set of medicinal qualities, are used in herbal treatments. Whether using decoctions, infusions, or essential oils, the extraction techniques are frequently age-old and tried-and-true. The effectiveness of these treatments has been more and more supported by modern science, which has also helped to clarify the processes by which different plant components work as healers.

The rise in popularity of herbal treatments coincides with a more general trend in society toward natural and ecological lifestyles. Herbal remedies present a compelling alternative to synthetic drugs for those looking for alternatives because of their minimal environmental impact and therapeutic potential.

CHAPTER TWO

COMPREHENDING PAIN AND SLEEP
THE SIGNIFICANCE OF PAIN CONTROL

Since pain management is essential to improving people's overall well-being, it is a vital component of healthcare. A person's quality of life can be greatly impacted by pain, whether it be acute or chronic, as it can have an impact not only on physical health but also on emotional and psychological well-being. Pain relief and the avoidance of potentially more serious health problems are two reasons why effective pain management is so important.

Chronic pain, if left ignored, can lead to a cascade of negative consequences, including limited mobility, impaired cognitive function, and higher stress levels. Thus, knowledge of and application of pain management techniques are essential elements of overall healthcare.

THE SIGNIFICANCE OF SLEEP FOR GENERAL WELFARE

It is impossible to overestimate the importance of sleep as a basic component of general well-being. Several factors related to both physical and mental health are directly impacted by the quantity and quality of sleep. Sustaining optimal cognitive performance, emotional stability, and immune system resilience requires getting enough good-quality sleep. Lack of sleep or poor quality of sleep can aggravate several health problems, such as immune system weakness, mood disorders, and difficulty concentrating. Therefore, encouraging a healthy and balanced lifestyle requires giving proper sleep hygiene a priority and resolving sleep-related issues.

RELATIONSHIP BETWEEN SLEEP AND PAIN

The delicate connection between sleep and pain emphasizes how complicated human physiology is. Sleep and pain are mutually reinforcing, with each having a significant impact on the other. Sleep habits can be disturbed by chronic pain, making it harder to fall asleep or stay asleep through the night. On the other hand, getting too little or poor quality sleep can make it harder to tolerate pain and make it feel worse. An individual's overall influence on their well-being may be exacerbated by this mutually reinforcing cycle of pain and sleep problems.

The relationship between pain and sleep is influenced by several physiological processes. An inability to smoothly transition between different stages of sleep might be caused by pain signals interfering with the regular sleep cycle. On the other hand, by making the neurological system more sensitive, sleep disturbances might increase the perception of pain. The fact that disorders including insomnia, restless legs syndrome, and sleep apnea are known to coexist with chronic pain issues highlights the complex link between the two.

Concurrently addressing pain and sleep-related problems is crucial for holistic treatment and better patient results. To end the cycle of pain and sleep disruptions, a multidisciplinary strategy involving medical therapies, lifestyle changes, and behavioral methods is frequently required. Physicians, physical therapists, and sleep specialists are among the healthcare providers who work together to create individualized treatment regimens that are tailored to each patient's specific needs. Healthcare professionals can help improve their patient's general health and quality of life by identifying and treating the link between pain and sleep.

CHAPTER THREE

TYPICAL REASONS FOR PAIN AND SLEEP ISSUES

CONDITIONS ASSOCIATED WITH CHRONIC PAIN

Chronic pain is defined as ongoing suffering that persists longer than the anticipated period of recovery. It may arise from several ailments, including back injuries, migraines, fibromyalgia, and arthritis. These illnesses frequently affect the neural system, which makes people more sensitive to pain sensations. One's quality of life can be negatively impacted by chronic pain, which can affect one's physical and mental health. Constant discomfort might cause sleep difficulties, which would then start a vicious cycle where pain gets worse and sleep issues get worse.

TYPES OF SLEEP DISORDERS

Conditions that disrupt regular sleep patterns fall under the broad category of sleep disorders. Having trouble falling or staying asleep is a common sleep problem known as insomnia. Another common problem is sleep apnea, which causes breathing pauses during the night, interfering with the natural sleep-wake cycle. The insatiable need to move the legs is a symptom of restless legs syndrome (RLS), which is frequently accompanied by uncomfortable feelings. Other sleep disorders include parasomnias, which include sleepwalking and night terrors, and narcolepsy, which is characterized by excessive daytime sleepiness. While the symptoms of each condition are unique, many of them have a reciprocal link with chronic pain.

INTERACTION BETWEEN PAIN AND SLEEP

There is a complicated and reciprocal relationship between pain and sleep. Because it can be uncomfortable and difficult to find a comfortable sleeping posture, chronic pain can interfere with sleep. In turn, sleep problems have the potential to intensify pain perception. The body's healing processes depend on sleep, and when it is disturbed, the pain tolerance may be lowered. Chronic pain can also be made worse by sleep deprivation, which can also lead to weariness, irritation, and mental distress.

Inflammatory processes are important for controlling pain and sleep. Chronic inflammation is a factor in pain and sleep-wake disturbance in conditions like arthritis. Furthermore, neurotransmitters involved in mood and pain management, such as norepinephrine and serotonin, also influence sleep regulation. Both sleep difficulties and chronic pain illnesses can be attributed to imbalances in these neurotransmitters.

Anxiety and stress are two psychological variables that can influence how pain and sleep interact. Emotional anguish brought on by chronic pain frequently causes sleep disruptions. On the other hand, insufficient sleep might worsen coping strategies and emotional control, which increases pain perception. Taking care of the psychological components of sleep difficulties and pain is essential to ending the cycle and enhancing general health.

There is a complex link between chronic pain syndromes and sleep difficulties. It is essential to comprehend the intricate relationship between pain and sleep to create successful treatment plans. People with chronic pain and sleep difficulties need comprehensive methods that address the psychological and physical components of these disorders to improve their quality of life.

CHAPTER FOUR

OVERVIEW OF HERBAL TREATMENTS

AN HISTORICAL VIEW ON HERBAL MEDICINE

Throughout history, herbal treatments have been used in many different nations and civilizations. Herbal therapy has long been the mainstay of treatment in many ancient societies. Many societies, including those of ancient Greece, Egypt, India, and China, gained a great deal of information about the therapeutic qualities of plants.

Herbal medicine was a deeply rooted part of traditional traditions, frequently entwined with spiritual beliefs. Historical records, such as the works of Hippocrates and the ancient Chinese pharmacopeia, attest to the application of particular herbs in the treatment of a variety of illnesses. This historical viewpoint emphasizes the continued applicability of herbal treatment and its crucial contribution to laying the groundwork for modern medical science.

THE EFFECTIVENESS AND SAFETY OF HERBAL REMEDIES

Research and examination into the effectiveness and safety of herbal treatments have not stopped. Although herbal therapy provides a natural and all-encompassing method of treatment, questions have been raised concerning possible interactions and negative effects of prescription drugs. When evaluating the efficacy and safety of herbal treatments, scientific research, and clinical trials are essential. The pharmacological characteristics of the active ingredients in plants, such as terpenes, flavonoids, and alkaloids, are investigated. Ensuring consistency and dependability in the effectiveness of herbal treatments is facilitated by standardizing herbal preparations and implementing quality control procedures. However, because there are so many different plant species and herbal formulations with different compositions, it is still difficult to create consistent recommendations.

INCLUDING HERBS IN CONTEMPORARY MEDICINE

Herbal therapies are becoming more and more popular in modern healthcare when combined with traditional medical procedures. A change toward a more patient-centered and comprehensive approach is reflected in this integration. Numerous medical experts are aware of the potential advantages of integrating herbal therapy with orthodox medicine to improve patient outcomes. Integrative medicine recognizes the importance of herbal medicines in supporting general well-being and promotes cooperation between traditional healthcare and complementary therapies. Studies investigate the interactions between pharmaceutical medications and herbal remedies to enhance treatment plans and enhance patient outcomes. The incorporation of herbal medicines into contemporary healthcare is a dynamic and developing field that has the potential to lead to a more all-encompassing approach to health and healing.

A thorough comprehension of the lasting importance of herbal medicine in medical procedures can be gained from its historical foundations. A more knowledgeable and evidence-based integration of herbal treatments into contemporary healthcare is made possible by the continuous investigation into their safety and effectiveness. Herbal medicine is changing, and when combined with traditional therapies, it represents a more all-encompassing strategy aimed at maximizing patient care and wellness. Herbal treatments are expected to become an increasingly important part of a wider range of healthcare practices as long as study and collaboration on the subject continue.

CHAPTER FIVE

HERBAL REMEDIES FOR PAIN

CURCUMIN AND TURMERIC

Due to their well-known strong anti-inflammatory qualities, turmeric and its key ingredient, curcumin, are well-liked options for natural pain management. For millennia, traditional medicine, especially Ayurveda, has employed turmeric to treat a wide range of illnesses. The primary bioactive component of turmeric, curcumin, is well-known for its capacity to block the body's inflammatory pathways.

According to research, curcumin may be useful in easing the pain brought on by inflammatory illnesses and conditions like arthritis. A comprehensive strategy for pain management may involve supplementing with turmeric or including it in one's diet.

GINGER

Another herb well-known for its analgesic and anti-inflammatory qualities is ginger. Some of its active ingredients, like gingerol, have shown analgesic properties. Traditional uses of ginger include pain relief from menstruation discomfort and osteoarthritis. Ginger can be an adaptable and affordable choice for anyone looking for herbal pain relief, whether it is drunk as a tea, added to food, or taken as a supplement.

WILLOW BARK

The bark of the white willow tree, which is used to make willow bark, has long been used in traditional medicine as a pain reliever. Salicin, the active component of willow bark, is comparable to aspirin's primary constituent. Because of this, willow bark's analgesic and anti-inflammatory qualities have been acknowledged. Willow bark can be a good natural pain reliever, while it might not be for everyone, especially for those who are allergic to aspirin.

BOSWELLIA

Indian frankincense, or Boswellia, is made from the resin of the Boswellia serrata tree. Boswellic acids, which are the active ingredients in boswellia, have anti-inflammatory properties that may help with pain management. Traditional Ayurvedic medicine has employed this plant for several inflammatory disorders, including arthritis. Supplements containing Boswellia are obtainable and could be incorporated into a comprehensive pain management strategy.

ARNICA

Because of its anti-inflammatory qualities, arnica, a perennial herb native to Europe and Siberia, has been applied topically. Arnica extracts are frequently used topically as creams, gels, or ointments to lessen the discomfort and swelling brought on by sprains, bruises, and tightness in the muscles. Arnica is generally safe to apply topically, but it's important to take the recommended quantity and avoid ingesting it.

ALTERNATIVE HERBAL REMEDIES

There are several additional herbal remedies for pain treatment in addition to the ones described above. For example, devil's claw has long been used to treat arthritis and lower back pain due to its anti-inflammatory qualities. Ginger, a related of turmeric, and cat's claw, another herbal treatment, are also known to have anti-inflammatory and pain-relieving properties. Meadowsweet, white willow bark, and St. John's Wort are other herbs that have been used traditionally for their analgesic qualities.

Before adding herbal therapies to a pain management regimen, people should exercise caution and see a healthcare provider, particularly if they are on medication or already have a medical problem. Herbs can provide natural pain treatment options, but there is a range in their safety and effectiveness, so using them wisely is crucial for general health.

CHAPTER SIX

HERBS TO HELP YOU SLEEP

ROOT OF VALERIAN

Popular for its ability to induce relaxation and ease sleeplessness, Valerian Root is a herb. Compounds in the root interact with the brain's gamma-aminobutyric acid (GABA) receptors to produce a relaxing effect. Valerian root is frequently used to aid those with sleep issues in herbal teas, pills, or tinctures. Numerous reports of better sleep quality have been made, yet research on its efficacy is still underway.

A PASSIONFLOWER

Another plant that may help you fall asleep is passionflower, which has long been used to treat insomnia and anxiety. Compounds in the plant may raise GABA levels in the brain, which would add to the calming effect. Studies have suggested that passionflower, which is often taken as a tea or supplement, can help induce sleep and lessen anxiety. To determine its long-term safety and efficacy, more study is necessary.

LAVENDER

Renowned for its pleasing aroma, lavender is often used in aromatherapy and is also known to aid with sleep. Lavender essential oil is thought to offer relaxing properties that can aid in promoting sleep and enhancing the quality of sleep. Lavender oil is a common ingredient in diffusers, sprays, and sleep routines that help people relax. Preliminary study indicates that lavender may improve sleep, but more studies are required.

LEMON BALM

A member of the mint family, lemon balm has long been used as a stress and anxiety reliever. Its potential as a sleep aid may be aided by its modest sedative qualities. Many people drink lemon balm tea, and research suggests that it may help lessen the symptoms of insomnia and enhance the quality of sleep. However, as with many herbal medicines, more investigation is needed to determine its efficacy and comprehend its mode of action.

ALTERNATIVE HERBAL REMEDIES

Apart from these widely recognized herbs, individuals experiment with several herbal alternatives as a means of promoting sleep. For example, chamomile is a well-liked option because of its relaxing qualities and mild sedative effects. A popular beverage before bed, chamomile tea is well-known for its calming effects on the body and mind. Herbs with the potential to promote sleep include ashwagandha, hops, and skullcap, among many others that people take into consideration.

While herbal medicines can provide a natural solution for sleep problems, it's crucial to remember that individual results may differ. It is advisable to speak with a healthcare provider before introducing herbs into a sleep pattern, particularly for people who take prescriptions that may mix with herbal supplements or have pre-existing health concerns. Achieving good sleep patterns also heavily depends on lifestyle choices like keeping a regular sleep schedule and establishing a comfortable sleeping environment.

HERBAL INFUSIONS AND TEAS: HERBAL FORMULATIONS AND RECIPES

For ages, herbal infusions and teas have been a crucial component of traditional medical systems, utilizing the medicinal qualities of diverse plants to enhance overall health and wellness. Herbal infusions are made by steeping fresh or dried herbs in hot water, allowing the water to draw out the therapeutic ingredients found in the plant material. This gentle extraction process is preferred because it is easy to use and works well to preserve the delicate components of herbs.

Herbal infusions are usually made by boiling water, adding the necessary herbs, and allowing the mixture to steep for a predetermined period. Depending on the desired medicinal benefits, different herbs can be used and steeping times can be adjusted.

For instance, teas made with peppermint and ginger are frequently used to help with digestion, while infusions of chamomile and lavender are recognized for their calming effects.

HERBAL TINCTURES

Herbal tinctures are a concentrated type of herbal medicine that is made by extracting and preserving the active ingredients of plants with alcohol or a combination of alcohol and water. The selected herbs are macerated and steeped in the alcohol solution for a considerable amount of time to create the tincture. This process guarantees a strong and durable herbal extract.

Because the alcohol in tinctures acts as a natural preservative, they have a longer shelf life than teas and infusions. They also offer herbal medicine in a convenient and doable form. Herbs that are frequently used in tinctures include milk thistle for liver health, valerian for relaxation, and echinacea for immunological support.

TOPICAL PLANT TREATMENTS

Herbs have long been prized for topical treatments in addition to their internal uses. Topical herbal preparations, which range from salves and ointments to creams and poultices, provide a targeted strategy to treat a variety of skin diseases and encourage recovery. Arnica is well-known for its capacity to relieve muscle discomfort, while calendula, with its anti-inflammatory qualities, is frequently utilized in salves to soothe inflamed skin.

Choosing plants with complementary qualities is essential to creating potent topical treatments. For instance, blending chamomile with lavender can result in a calming and anti-inflammatory mixture. The selection of carrier oils and other components, like shea butter or beeswax, increases the herbal mixtures' capacity for medicinal effects.

BLENDING HERBS TO GET OPTIMAL RESULTS

A key idea in herbal therapy is the synergy of herbs, which occurs when the combined effects of various plants improve the overall therapeutic outcome. Herbs can enhance one another's effects when they are thoughtfully chosen and blended, producing a more potent and well-rounded treatment. This strategy is especially noticeable in formulations meant to address complicated health problems.

For example, mixing turmeric and black pepper increases the absorption of curcumin, the molecule that gives turmeric its anti-inflammatory properties. Herbalists frequently create formulations that address several facets of a health issue by drawing on their understanding of the characteristics of each herb.

CHAPTER SEVEN

COMBINING CONVENTIONAL MEDICINE WITH HERBAL THERAPIES

ASSISTED BY HEALTHCARE PROVIDERS

Patients, healthcare professionals, and herbal practitioners must work together to integrate herbal therapy with mainstream medicine. To guarantee the patient's safety and wellbeing throughout this relationship, effective communication and transparency are crucial. Healthcare professionals, including as doctors and nurses, are essential in helping patients integrate into their new lives, informing them of the advantages and disadvantages, and keeping an eye on their general well-being.

Understanding a patient's medical history, current therapies, and any lingering health concerns requires open communication between the patient and healthcare providers. Healthcare professionals are better equipped to decide whether to include herbal medicines in the overall treatment plan thanks to this collaboration. Additionally, it makes knowledge exchange between traditional medicine and herbal remedies possible, which promotes a more thorough and all-encompassing approach to patient care.

MEDICATIONS AND POSSIBLE INTERACTIONS

Taking into account possible drug interactions is a crucial part of combining herbal remedies with traditional medicine. Bioactive chemicals found in herbal supplements have the potential to interact with prescription medications, either causing unwanted side effects or altering their efficacy. Healthcare professionals must be aware of these interactions and carefully consider whether herbal medicines and prescription drugs are compatible.

Some herbs may affect how medications are metabolized in the liver, which can affect how well the pharmaceuticals are absorbed, distributed, and eliminated from the body.

A deep understanding of pharmacology and herbal medicine is necessary to comprehend these interactions. To minimize side effects and maximize the therapeutic benefits of traditional treatments, medical professionals must ask patients about everything they take in, including herbal supplements. Herbal Supplements as Complementary Therapies: When combined with traditional medicine, herbal supplements are frequently seen as complementary therapies. They can be helpful in the management of several medical disorders, including stress, inflammation, and chronic pain. Herbal supplements and pharmaceutical medications can work in concert to improve treatment outcomes overall and give patients a more all-encompassing approach to their well-being.

Herbal supplements may be used by patients to treat particular symptoms, enhance general health, or lessen the negative effects of prescription drugs. By enabling people to actively engage in their healthcare decisions, the use of herbal remedies can support a patient-centered care model.

Nonetheless, while considering herbal supplements as a part of their treatment plan, healthcare providers must emphasize to patients the value of making educated decisions and the necessity of expert supervision and evidence-based information.

Patients and healthcare professionals must work together to successfully incorporate herbal medicines with mainstream medication. This method necessitates open communication, careful evaluation of any drug interactions, and acknowledgment of herbal supplements as supplemental therapy. By promoting collaboration between traditional medicine and herbal remedies, medical practitioners can provide patients with more individualized and comprehensive care, which will ultimately improve their general health.

CHAPTER EIGHT

LIFESTYLE AND PROPER SLEEP PRACTICES

THE VALUE OF MAKING HEALTHY LIFESTYLE DECISIONS

Making healthy lifestyle choices is essential to total well-being, which goes beyond physical health to include mental and emotional well-being. Adopting a healthy lifestyle requires a multifaceted strategy that includes stress reduction, regular exercise, a balanced diet, and enough sleep. Our daily decisions have a significant impact on our general health, impacting not only our physical and mental well-being but also our resilience and emotional equilibrium.

ESTABLISHING A CALM SLEEP ENVIRONMENT

A vital part of keeping up a healthy lifestyle is making sure you get enough good sleep by practicing good sleep hygiene. Sleep is essential for maintaining emotional control, cognitive abilities, and physical healing.

Promoting healthy sleep requires creating a calm and comfortable sleeping environment. This entails maximizing elements like lighting, noise levels, and room temperature to produce a cozy and peaceful environment that promotes sleep.

By reducing disturbances and establishing a relaxing environment, people can increase the quality of their sleep, which in turn improves their general health.

THE EFFECTS OF EXERCISE ON PAIN AND SLEEP

Another essential component of a healthy lifestyle is exercise, which has benefits that go beyond improved physical fitness. Improved sleep duration and quality have been associated with regular physical activity. Better sleep patterns can result from moderate-intensity cardiovascular exercise, such as brisk walking or cycling. Exercise helps control stress hormones and encourages the release of endorphins, which are organic mood enhancers. These effects assist inducing a relaxed state of mind that is favorable for sleeping.

Moreover, there is a considerable correlation between exercise, discomfort, and sleep. Chronic pain can severely interfere with sleep, creating a vicious cycle in which pain gets worse when sleep is disrupted, and pain gets worse when sleep is disrupted even more.

Exercise regularly has been demonstrated to help people with chronic pain disorders sleep better and reduce their symptoms.

Exercise's physiological and psychological advantages support both the general promotion of restful sleep and pain management.

As healthy lifestyle choices are the cornerstone of mental, emotional, and physical well-being, their significance cannot be emphasized. This lifestyle places a strong emphasis on the importance of good sleep hygiene habits and the creation of a peaceful sleeping environment.

Furthermore, realizing how exercise affects pain management and sleep quality emphasizes how these two facets of healthy living are intertwined. People can cultivate a lifestyle that supports their well-being and encourages deep, rejuvenating sleep by adopting holistic practices and making educated decisions.

CHAPTER NINE

MIND-BODY METHODS FOR PAIN MANAGEMENT AND SLEEP

MEDITATION AND MINDFULNESS

These two approaches have become more well-known for their effectiveness in treating pain and sleep-related disorders. Although these methods have their roots in antiquated customs, they are nevertheless widely used in modern medicine. Training the mind to attain a state of heightened awareness and focused concentration is the goal of meditation. Being present in the moment without passing judgment is emphasized by mindfulness, which is a crucial component of meditation.

According to research, frequent meditation can improve one's perception of pain by changing the way the brain interprets pain signals. For instance, mindfulness helps people to notice their feelings without being emotionally involved, which promotes a more adaptable way to deal with discomfort. Additionally, the relaxing effects of meditation serve to enhance the quality of sleep by reducing tension and anxiety, which are frequently the causes of sleep disturbances.

Even for little periods, meditating every day has the potential to improve sleep quality and lessen chronic pain. Clinical settings have effectively employed mindfulness-based stress reduction (MBSR) programs, which incorporate meditation practices, to address pain management and sleep issues.

YOGA FOR PAIN RELIEF AND SLEEP

Yoga is an age-old Indian practice that has developed into a multifaceted mind-body method that significantly reduces pain and improves sleep. Yoga's holistic approach integrates breathing exercises (pranayama), physical postures (asanas), and meditation to improve health in all aspects.

Gentle stretches and movements that target tense areas are frequently the focus of yoga sequences created specifically with pain reduction in mind. These exercises not only help to improve strength and flexibility but also to lessen chronic pain issues and reduce muscular stiffness. It has been demonstrated that incorporating restorative yoga postures into nighttime rituals can help promote relaxation and get the body ready for sound sleep.

Yoga's meditative elements are very important for relieving stress, increasing mental relaxation, and quieting the mind. Yoga creates a mind-body connection through the integration of awareness into movement, which can have a beneficial effect on how pain is perceived and help create a more peaceful sleeping environment.

BREATHING TECHNIQUES

Breathing exercises sometimes referred to as diaphragmatic or deep breathing, are an essential part of mind-body methods for pain relief and better sleep. These breathing exercises focus on deliberate and regulated breathing patterns to encourage the body's natural relaxing response.

When using a deep breathing technique, the breath is gradually exhaled via pursed lips after being inhaled slowly through the nose and allowed to fill the lungs. By purposefully concentrating on the breath, one can induce a calming mood and lessen the body's reactions to stress and discomfort by stimulating the parasympathetic nervous system.

Controlled breathing can help people focus on things other than their pain and improve their coping skills when it comes to managing their pain. Additionally, adding breathing exercises to pre-sleep rituals helps to calm the mind and create a peaceful atmosphere that supports sound sleep.